The Definitive Dash Diet Recipes Guide for Beginners

Affordable Soups and Salads Recipes to Get Back in Shape and Enjoy your Diet

I0222583

Naomi Hudson

Table of contents

Leek and Cauliflower Soup

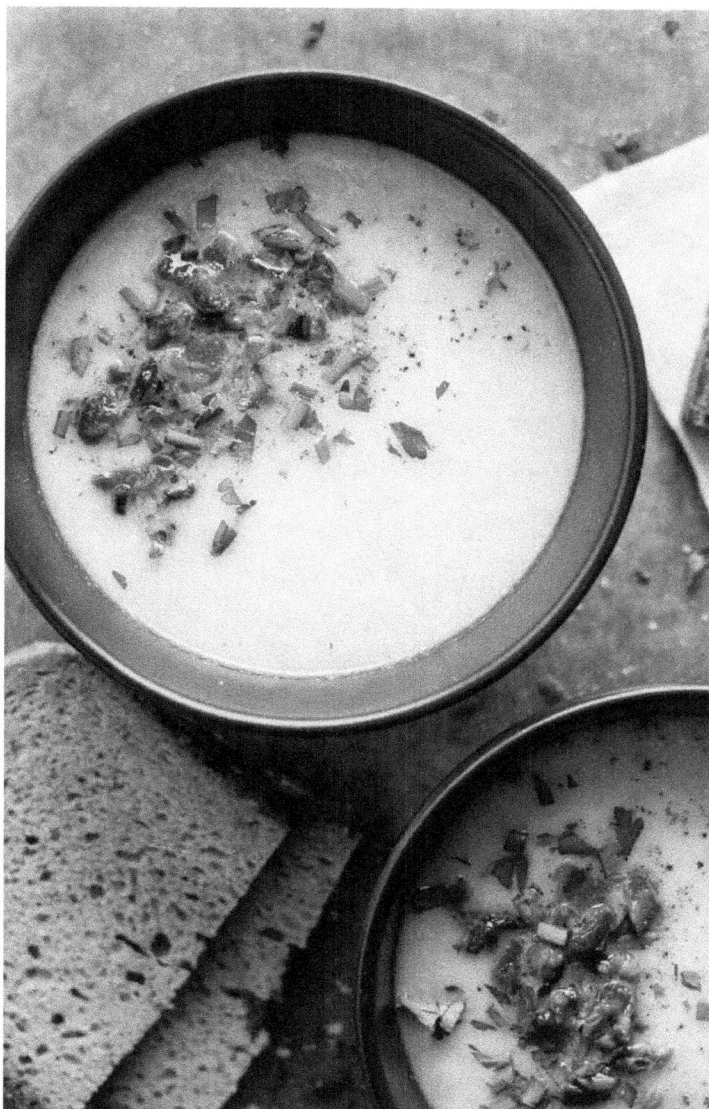

Serving: 6

Prep Time: 10 minutes

Cook Time: 40 minutes

Ingredients:

- 3 cups cauliflower, riced

- 1 bay leaf

- 1 teaspoon herbs de Provence

- 2 garlic cloves, peeled and diced

- ½ cup coconut milk

- 2 ½ cups vegetable stock

- 1 tablespoon coconut oil

- ½ teaspoon cracked pepper

- 1 leek, chopped

How To:

1. Take a pot, heat oil into it.

2. Sauté the leeks in the oil for 5 minutes.
3. Add the garlic and then stir-cook for another minute.

4.   Add all the remaining ingredients and mix them well.
5.   Cook for 30 minutes.
6.   Stir occasionally.
7.   Blend the soup until smooth by using an immersion blender.

8.   Serve hot and enjoy!

Nutrition (Per Serving)

Calories: 90

Fat: 7g

Carbohydrates: 4g

Protein: 2g

Dreamy Zucchini Bowl

Serving: 4

Prep Time: 10 minutes

Cook Time: 20 minutes

Ingredients:

- 1 onion, chopped

- 3 zucchini, cut into medium chunks

- 2 tablespoons coconut almond milk

- 2 garlic cloves, minced

- 4 cups vegetable stock

- 2 tablespoons coconut oil

- Pinch of sunflower seeds

- Black pepper to taste

How To:

1. Take a pot and place it over medium heat.

2. Add oil and let it heat up.
3. Add zucchini, garlic, onion and stir.
4. Cook for 5 minutes.
5. Add stock, sunflower seeds, pepper and stir.
6. Bring to a boil and reduce heat.
7. Simmer for 20 minutes.
8. Remove from heat and add coconut almond milk.

9. Use an immersion blender until smooth.
10. Ladle into soup bowls and serve.

11. Enjoy!

Nutrition (Per Serving)

Calories: 160

Fat: 2g

Carbohydrates: 4g

Protein: 7g

Cold Crab and Watermelon Soup

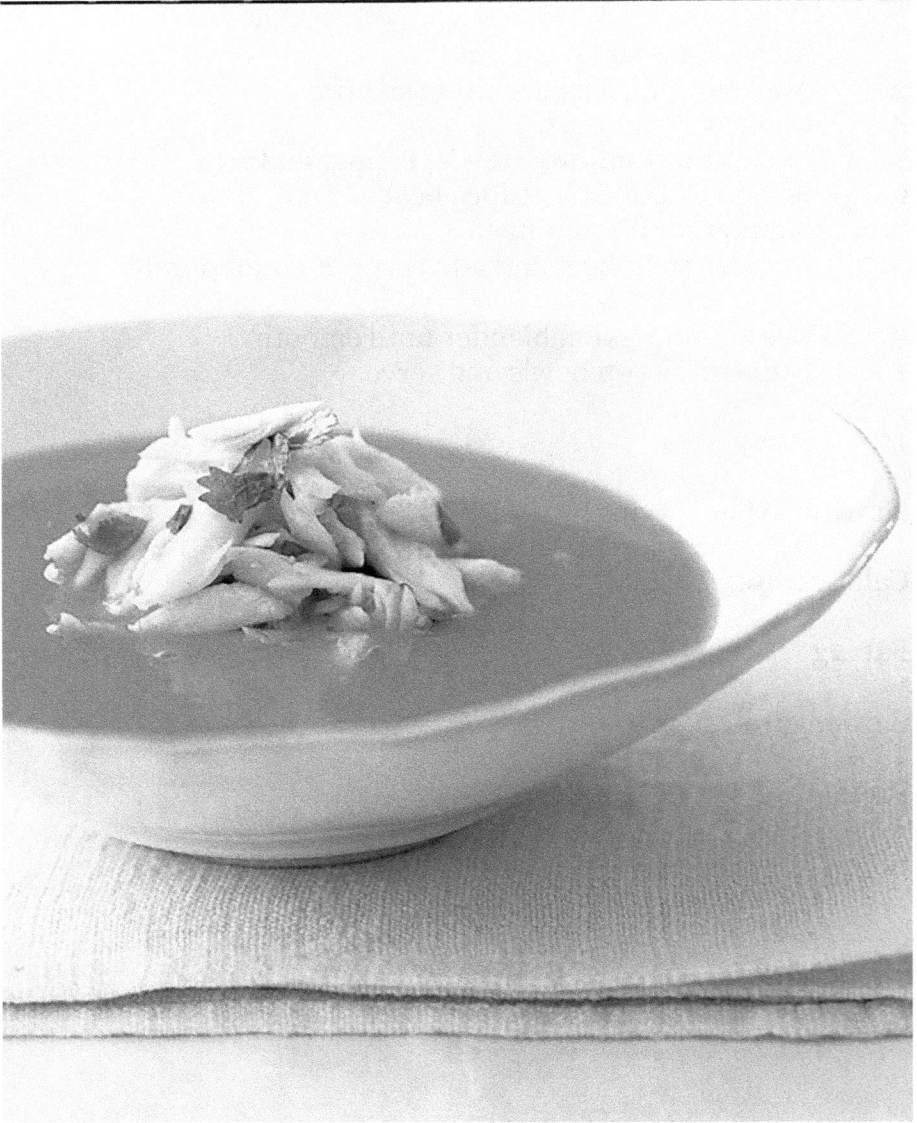

Serving: 4

Prep Time: 10 minutes + chill time

Cook Time: nil

Ingredients:

- ¼ cup basil, chopped

- 2 pounds tomatoes

- 5 cups watermelon, cubed

- ¼ cup wine vinegar

- 2 garlic cloves, minced

- 1 zucchini, chopped

- Pepper to taste

- 1 cup crabmeat

How To:

1.   Take your blender and add tomatoes, basil, vinegar, 4 cups watermelon, garlic, 1/3 cup oil, pepper and pulse well.

2.   Transfer to fridge and chill for 1 hour.
3.   Divide into bowls and add zucchini, crab and remaining watermelon.

4.   Serve and enjoy!

Nutrition (Per Serving)

Calories: 121

Fat: 3g

Carbohydrates: 4g

Protein: 8g

Paleo Lemon and Garlic Soup

Serving: 4

Prep Time: 10 minutes

Cook Time: 10 minutes

Ingredients:

- 6 cups shellfish stock

- 1 tablespoon garlic, minced

- 1 tablespoon coconut oil, melted

- 2 whole eggs

- ½ cup lemon juice

- Pinch of salt

- White pepper to taste

- 1 tablespoon arrowroot powder

- Finely chopped cilantro for serving

How To:

1.   Heat up a pot with oil over medium high heat.

2.   Add garlic, stir cook for 2 minutes.
3.   Add stock (reserve ½ cup for later use).

4.   Stir and bring mix to a simmer.

5.   Take a bowl and add eggs, sea salt, pepper, reserved stock, lemon juice and arrowroot.
6.   Whisk well.
7.   Pour in to the soup and cook for a few minutes.
8.   Ladle soup into bowls and serve with chopped cilantro.
9.   Enjoy!

Nutrition (Per Serving)

Calories: 135

Fat: 3g

Carbohydrates: 12g

Protein: 8

Brussels Soup

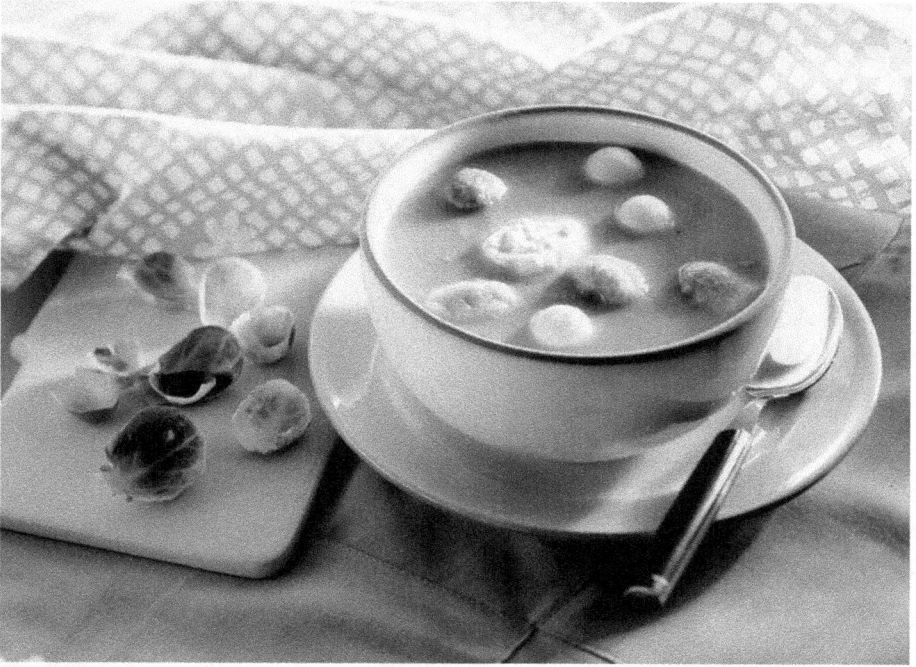

Serving: 4

Prep Time: 10 minutes

Cook Time: 20 minutes

Ingredients:

- 2 tablespoons olive oil
- 1 yellow onion, chopped

- 2 pounds Brussels sprouts, trimmed and halved

- 4 cups chicken stock

- ¼ cup coconut cream

How To:

1. Take a pot and place it over medium heat.

2. Add oil and let it heat up.
3. Add onion and stir-cook for 3 minutes.
4. Add Brussels sprouts and stir, cook for 2 minutes.
5. Add stock and black pepper, stir and bring to a simmer.
6. Cook for 20 minutes more.
7. Use an immersion blender to make the soup creamy.
8. Add coconut cream and stir well.

9. Ladle into soup bowls and serve.

10. Enjoy!

Nutrition (Per Serving)

Calories: 200

Fat: 11g

Carbohydrates: 6g

Protein: 11g

Spring Soup and Poached Egg

Serving: 4

Prep Time: 5 minutes

Cook Time: 15 minutes

Ingredients:

- 2 whole eggs

- 32 ounces chicken broth

- 1 head romaine lettuce, chopped

How To:

1.   Bring the chicken broth to a boil.

2.   Reduce the heat and poach the 2 eggs in the broth for 5 minutes.

3.   Take two bowls and transfer the eggs into a separate bowl.
4.   Add chopped romaine lettuce into the broth and cook for a few minutes.
5.   Serve the broth with lettuce into the bowls.
6.   Enjoy!

Nutrition (Per Serving)

Calories: 150

Fat: 5g

Carbohydrates: 6g

Protein: 16g

Lobster Bisque

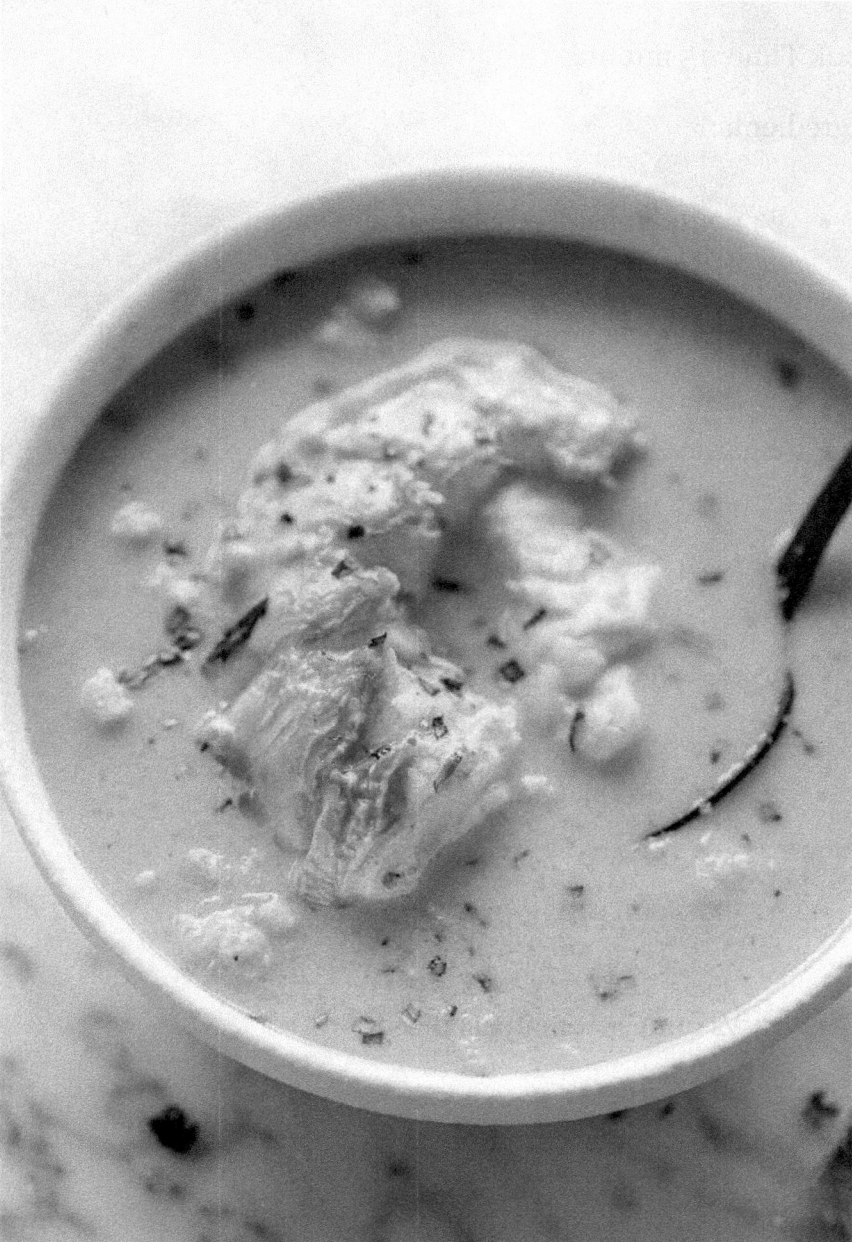

Serving: 4

Prep Time: 10 minutes

Cook Time: 15 minutes

Ingredients:

- ¾ pound lobster, cooked and lobster

- 4 cups chicken broth

- 2 garlic cloves, chopped

- ¼ teaspoon pepper

- ½ teaspoon paprika

- 1 yellow onion, chopped

- ½ teaspoon salt

- 14 ½ ounces tomatoes, diced

- 1 tablespoon coconut oil

- 1 cup low fat cream

How To:

1.   Take a stockpot and add the coconut oil over medium heat.

2.   Then sauté the garlic and onion for 3 to 5 minutes.
3.   Add diced tomatoes, spices and chicken broth and bring to a boil.

4.   Reduce to a simmer, then simmer for about 10 minutes.
5.   Add the warmed heavy cream to the soup.
6.   Blend the soup till creamy by using an immersion blender.
7.   Stir in cooked lobster.
8.   Serve and enjoy!

Nutrition (Per Serving)

Calories: 180

Fat: 11g

Carbohydrates: 6g

Protein: 16g

Tomato Bisque

Serving: 4

Prep Time: 10 minutes

Cook Time: 40 minutes

Ingredients:

- 4 cups chicken broth

- 1 cup low fat cream

- 1 teaspoon thyme dried

- 3 cups canned whole, peeled tomatoes

- 2 tablespoons almond butter

- 3 garlic cloves, peeled

- Pepper as needed

How To:

1.   Take a stockpot and first add the butter to the bottom of a stockpot.

2.   Then add all the ingredients except heavy cream into it.
3.   Bring to a boil.
4.   Simmer for 40 minutes.
5.   Warm the heavy cream and stir into the soup.
6.   Serve and enjoy!

Nutrition (Per Serving)

Calories: 141

Fat: 12g

Carbohydrates: 4g

Protein: 4g

Chipotle Chicken Chowder

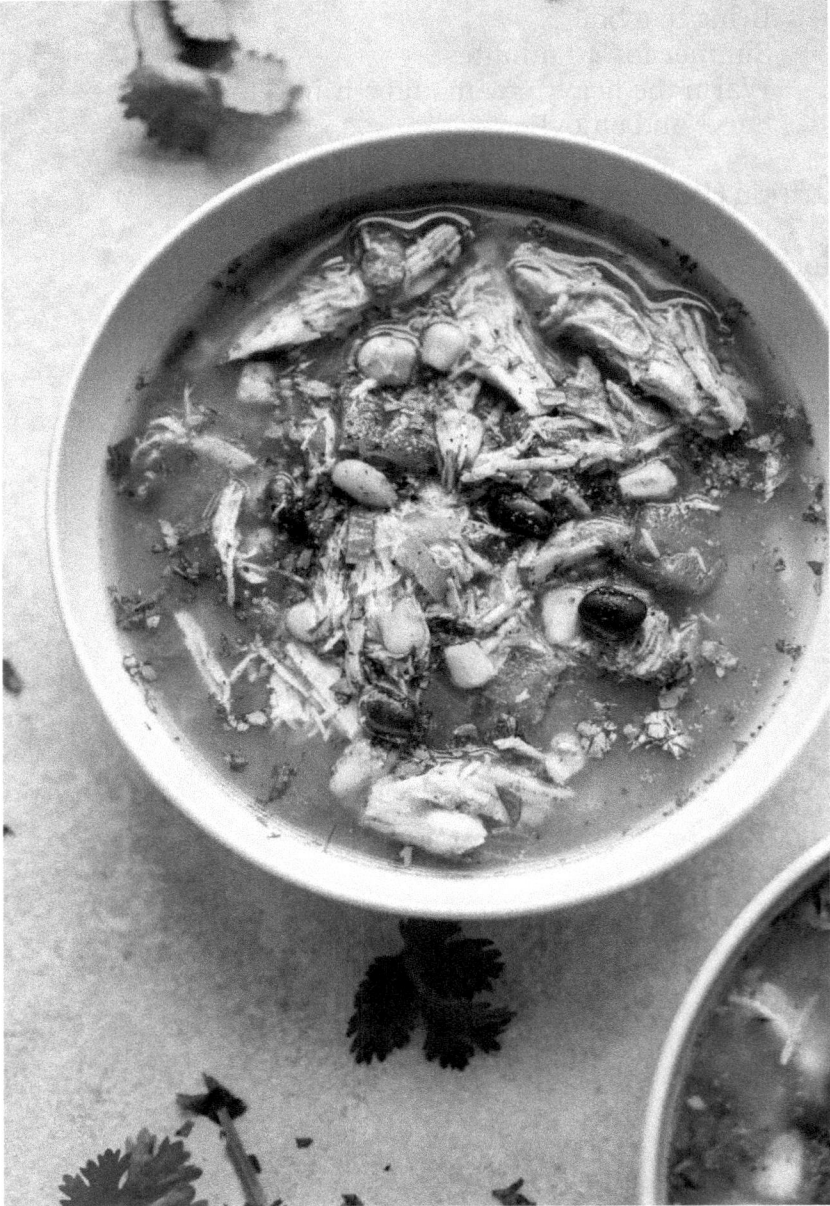

Serving: 4

Prep Time: 10 minutes

Cook Time: 23 minutes

Ingredients:

- 1 medium onion, chopped

- 2 garlic cloves, minced

- 6 bacon slices, chopped

- 4 cups jicama, cubed
- 3 cups chicken stock

- 1 teaspoon salt

- 2 cups low-fat, cream1 tablespoon olive oil

- 2 tablespoons fresh cilantro, chopped

- 1 ¼ pounds chicken, thigh boneless, cut into 1 inch chunks
  ½ teaspoon pepper

- 1 chipotle pepper, minced

How To:

1.   Heat olive oil over medium heat in a large sized saucepan, add bacon.

2.   Cook until crispy, add onion, garlic, and jicama.
3.   Cook for 7 minutes, add chicken stock and chicken.
4.   Bring to a boil and reduce temperature to low.
5.   Simmer for 10 minutes
6.   Season with salt and pepper.
7.   Add heavy cream and chipotle, simmer for 5 minutes.
8.   Sprinkle chopped cilantro and serve, enjoy!

Nutrition (Per Serving)

Calories: 350

Fat: 22g

Carbohydrates: 8g

Protein: 22g

Bay Scallop Chowder

Serving: 4

Prep Time: 10 minutes

Cook Time: 18 minutes

Ingredients:

- 1 medium onion, chopped

- 2 ½ cups chicken stock

- 4 slices bacon, chopped

- 3 cups daikon radish, chopped

- ½ teaspoon dried thyme

- 2 cups low-fat cream

- 1 tablespoon almond butter

- Pepper to taste

- 1 pound bay scallops

How To:

1.   Heat olive over medium heat in a large sized saucepan, add bacon and cook until crisp, add onion and daikon radish.

2.   Cook for 5 minutes, add chicken stock.
3.   Simmer for 8 minutes, season with salt and pepper, thyme.
4. Add heavy cream, bay scallops, simmer for 4 minutes
4.   Serve and enjoy!

Nutrition (Per Serving)

Calories: 307

Fat: 22g

Carbohydrates: 7g

Protein: 22g

Salmon and Vegetable Soup

Serving: 4

Prep Time: 10 minutes

Cook Time: 22 minutes

Ingredients:

- 2 tablespoons extra-virgin olive oil

- 1 leek, chopped

- 1 red onion, chopped

- Pepper to taste

- 2 carrots, chopped

- 4 cups low stock vegetable stock

- 4 ounces salmon, skinless and boneless, cubed ½ cup coconut cream

- 1 tablespoon dill, chopped

How To:

1.   Take a pan and place it over medium heat, add leek, onion, stir and cook for 7 minutes.

2.   Add pepper, carrots, stock and stir.
3.   Boil for 10 minutes.
4.   Add salmon, cream, dill and stir.
5.   Boil for 5-6 minutes.
6.   Ladle into bowls and serve.
7.   Enjoy!

Nutrition (Per Serving)

Calories: 240

Fat: 4g

Carbohydrates: 7g

Protein: 12g

Garlic Tomato Soup

Serving: 4

Prep Time: 15 minutes

Cook Time: 15 minutes

Ingredients:

- Roma tomatoes, chopped

- 1 cup tomatoes, sundried

- 2 tablespoons coconut oil

- 5 garlic cloves, chopped

- 14 ounces coconut milk

- 1 cup vegetable broth

- Pepper to taste

- Basil, for garnish

How To:

1.   Take a pot, heat oil into it.

2.   Sauté the garlic in it for ½ minute.

3.   Mix in the Roma tomatoes and cook for 8-10 minutes.

4.   Stir occasionally.
5.   Add in the rest of the ingredients, except the basil, and stir well.

6.   Cover the lid and cook for 5 minutes.
7.   Let it cool.
8.   Blend the soup until smooth by using an immersion blender.
9.   Garnish with basil.
10.   Serve and enjoy!

Nutrition (Per Serving)

Calories: 240

Fat: 23g

Carbohydrates: 16g

Protein: 7g

Melon Soup

Serving: 4

Prep Time:6 minutes

Cook Time: Nil

Ingredients:

- 4 cups casaba melon, seeded and cubed

- 1 tablespoon fresh ginger, grated

- ¾ cup coconut milk Juice of 2 limes

How To:

Add the lime juice, coconut milk, casaba melon, ginger and salt into your blender.

Blend for 1-2 minutes until you get a smooth mixture.

Serve and enjoy!

Nutrition (Per Serving)

Calories: 134

Fat: 9g

Carbohydrates: 13g

Protein: 2g

Spring Salad

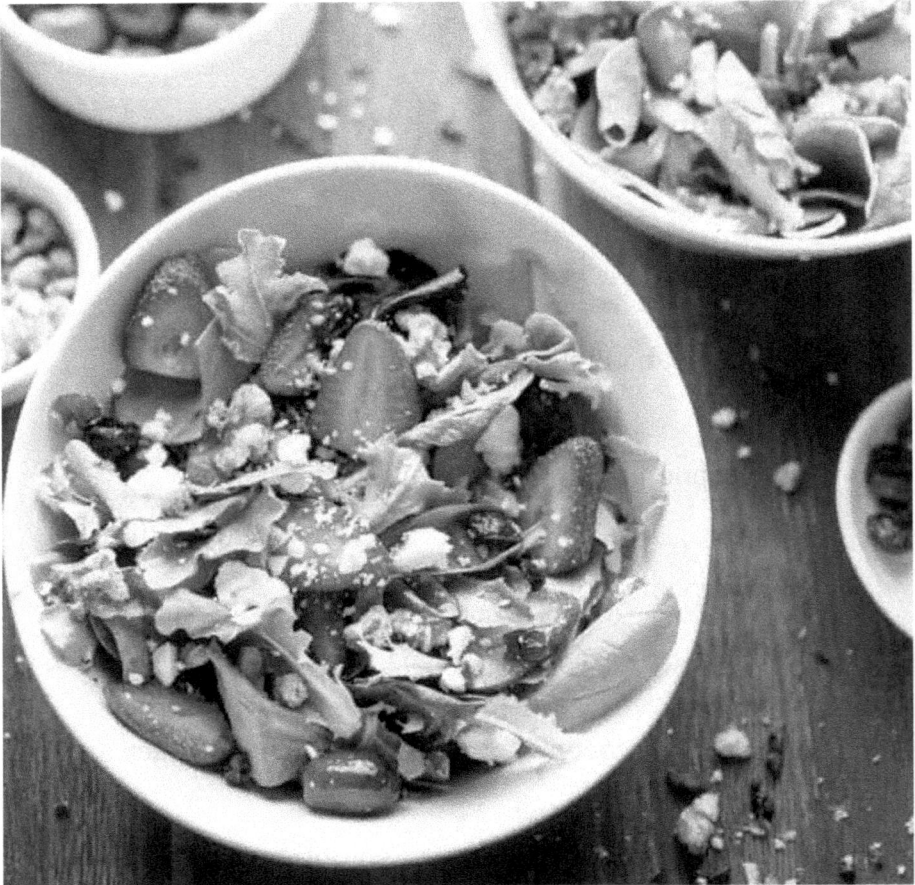

Serving: 2

Prep Time: 10-15 minutes

Cook Time: 0 minutes

Ingredients:

- 2 ounces mixed green vegetables

- 3 tablespoons roasted pine nuts

- 2 tablespoons 5-minute 5 Keto Raspberry Vinaigrette

- 2 tablespoons shaved Parmesan

- 2 slices bacon

Pepper as required

How To:

1.   Take a cooking pan and add bacon, cook the bacon until crispy.

2.   Take a bowl and add the salad ingredients and mix well, add crumbled bacon into the salad.
3.   Mix well.
4.   Dress it with your favorite dressing.
5.   Enjoy!

Nutrition (Per Serving)

Calories: 209

Fat: 17g

Net Carbohydrates: 10g

Protein: 4g

Hearty Orange and Onion Salad

Serving: 2

Prep Time: 10 minutes

Cook Time: nil

Ingredients:

6 large oranges

- 3 tablespoons red wine vinegar

- 6 tablespoons olive oil

- 1 teaspoon dried oregano

- 1 red onion, thinly sliced

- 1 cup olive oil

- ¼ cup fresh chives, chopped Ground black pepper

How To:

1.   Peel orange and cut into 4-5 crosswise slices.

2.   Transfer orange to shallow dish.

3. Drizzle vinegar, olive oil on top.
4. Sprinkle oregano.
5. Toss well to mix.
6. Chill for 30 minutes and arrange sliced onion and black olives on top.
7. Sprinkle more chives and pepper.
8. Serve and enjoy!

Nutrition (Per Serving)

Calories: 120

Fat: 6g

Carbohydrates: 20g

Protein: 2g

Ground Beef Bell Peppers

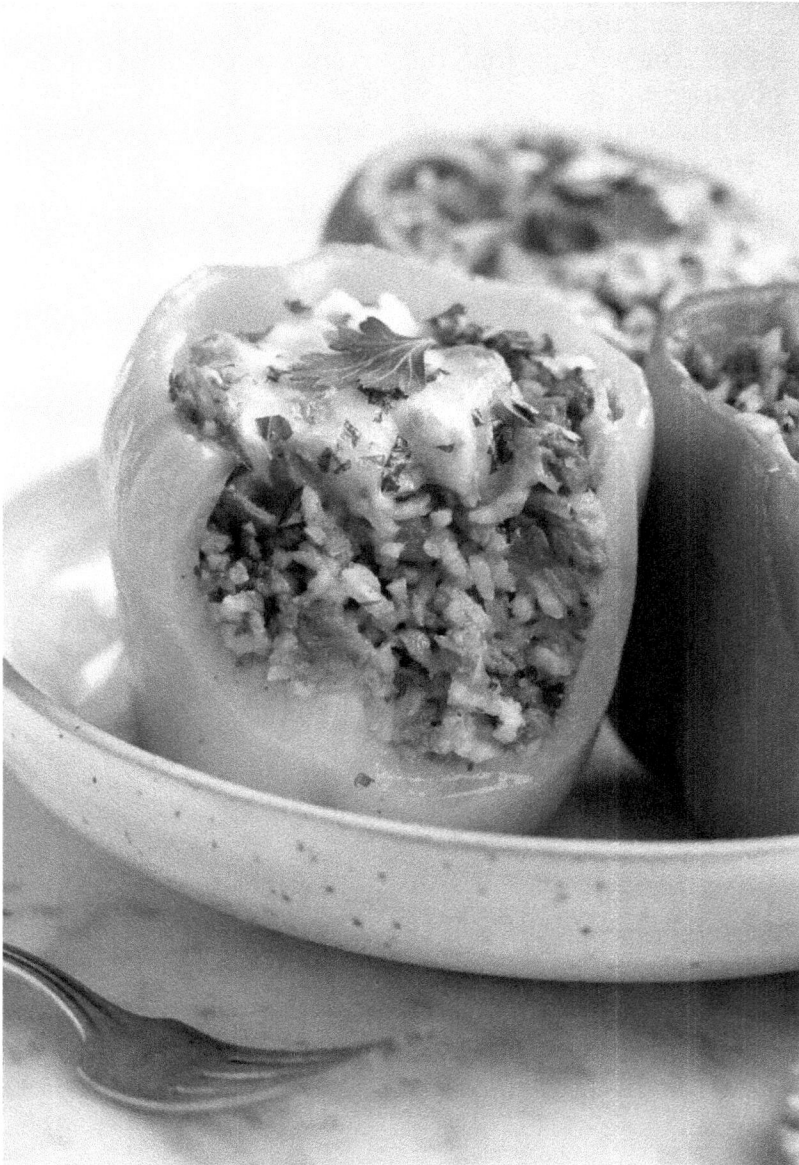

Serving: 3

Prep Time: 10 minutes

Cook Time: 10 minutes

Ingredients:

- 1 onion, chopped

- 2 tablespoons coconut oil

- 1 pound ground beef

- 1 red bell pepper, diced

- 2 cups spinach, chopped

- Pepper to taste

How To:

1. Take a skillet and place it over medium heat.

2. Add onion and cook until slightly browned.
3. Add spinach and ground beef.
4. Stir fry until done.
5. Take the mixture and fill up the bell peppers.
6. Serve and enjoy!

Nutrition (Per Serving)

Calories: 350

Fat: 23g

Carbohydrates: 4g

Protein: 28g

A Turtle Friend Salad

Serving: 6

Prep Time: 5 minutes

Cook Time: 5 minutes

Ingredients:

- 1 Romaine lettuce, chopped

- 3 Roma tomatoes, diced

- 1 English cucumber, diced

- 1 small red onion, diced

- ½ cup parsley, chopped

- 2 tablespoons virgin olive oil

- ½ large lemon, juice

- 1 teaspoon garlic powder

- Sunflower seeds and pepper to taste

How To:

1.   Wash the vegetables thoroughly under cold water.

2.   Prepare them by chopping, dicing or mincing as needed.
3.   Take a large salad bowl and transfer the prepped veggies.
4.   Add vegetable oil, olive oil, lemon juice, and spice.
5.   Toss well to coat.
6.   Serve chilled if preferred.
7.   Enjoy!

Nutrition (Per Serving)

Calories: 200

Fat: 8g

Carbohydrates: 18g

Protein: 10g

Avocado and Cilantro Mix

Serving: 2

Prep Time: 10 minutes

Cook Time: nil

Ingredients:

2 avocados, peeled, pitted and diced

- 1 sweet onion, chopped

- 1 green bell pepper, chopped

- 1 large ripe tomato, chopped

- ¼ cup of fresh cilantro, chopped

- ½ lime, juiced

- Sunflower seeds and pepper as needed

How To:

1.   Take a medium sized bowl and add onion, tomato, avocados, bell pepper, lime and cilantro.

2. Give the whole mixture a toss.

3. Season accordingly and serve chilled.
4. Enjoy!

Nutrition (Per Serving)

Calories: 126

Fat: 10g

Carbohydrates: 10g

Protein: 2g

Exceptional Watercress and Melon Salad

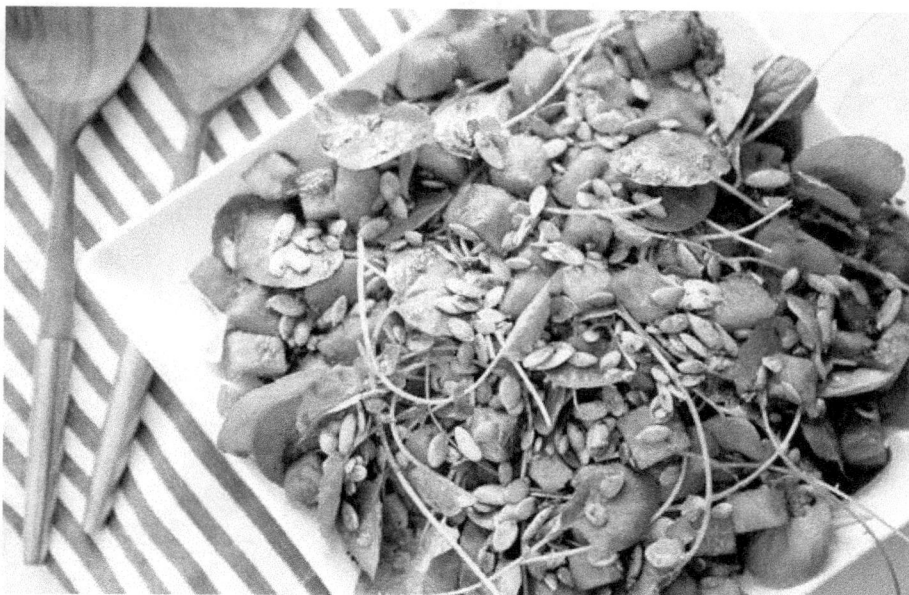

Serving: 4

Prep Time: 15 minutes

Cook Time: 20 minutes

Ingredients:

- 3 tablespoons lime juice

- 1 teaspoon date paste

- 1 teaspoon fresh ginger root, minced

- ¼ cup vegetable oil

- 2 bunch watercress, chopped

- 2 ½ cups watermelon, cubed

- 2 ½ cups cantaloupe, cubed

- 1/3 cup almonds, toasted and sliced

How To:

1.   Take a large sized bowl and add lime juice, ginger, date paste.

2.   Whisk well and add oil.
3.   Season with pepper and sunflower seeds.
4.   Add watercress, watermelon.
5.   Toss well
6.   Transfer to a serving bowl and garnish with sliced almonds.

7.   Enjoy!

Nutrition (Per Serving)

Calories: 274

Fat: 20g

Carbohydrates: 21g

Protein: 7g

Zucchini and Onions Platter

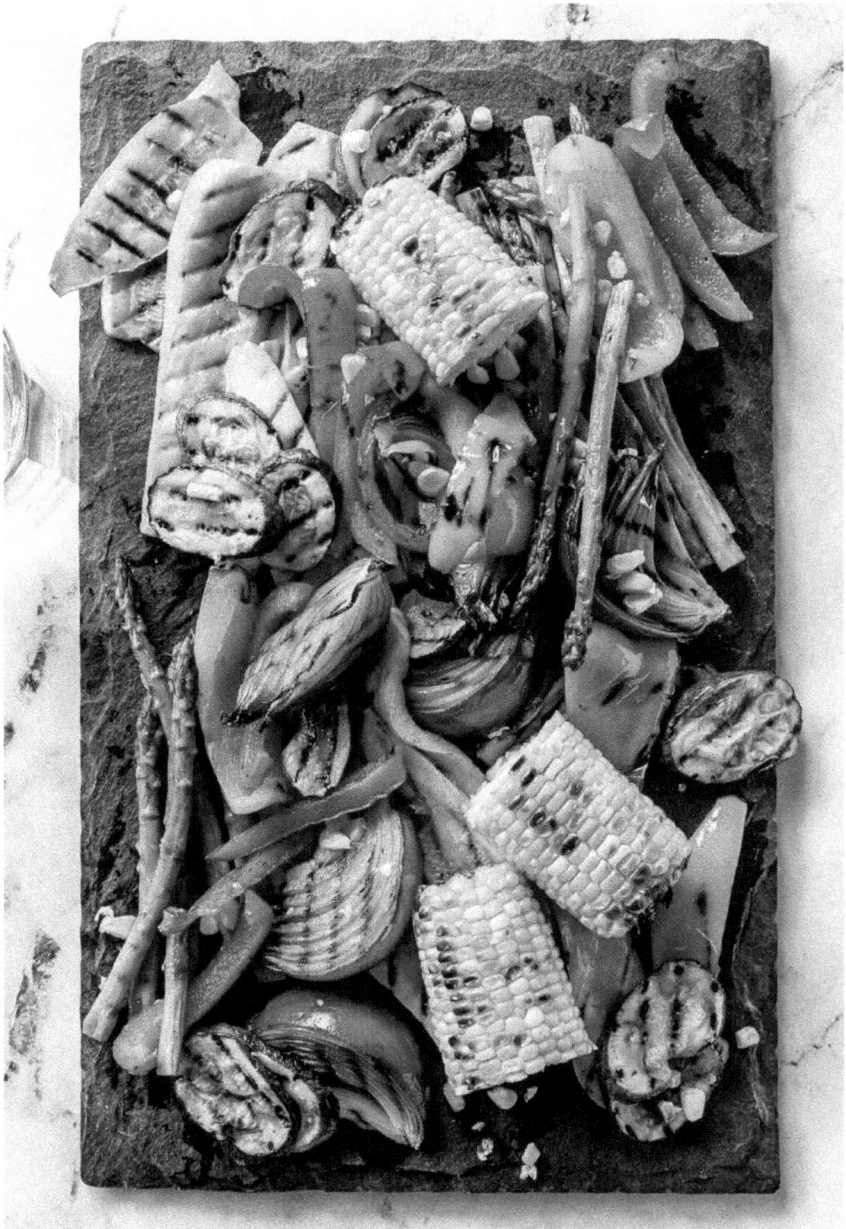

Serving: 4

Prep Time: 15 minutes

Cook Time: 45 minutes

Ingredients:

- 3 large zucchini, julienned

- 1 cup cherry tomatoes, halved

- ½ cup basil

- 2 red onions, thinly sliced

- ¼ teaspoon sunflower seeds

- 1 teaspoon cayenne pepper

- 2 tablespoons lemon juice

How To:

1.   Create zucchini Zoodles by using a vegetable peeler and shaving the zucchini with peeler lengthwise until you get to the core and seeds.
2.   Turn zucchini and repeat until you have long strips.
3.   Discard seeds.
4.   Lay strips in cutting board and slice lengthwise to your desired thickness.

5. Mix Zoodles in a bowl alongside onion, basil, tomatoes and toss.

6. Sprinkle sunflower seeds and cayenne pepper on top.
7. Drizzle lemon juice.
8. Serve and enjoy!

Nutrition (Per Serving)

Calories: 156

Fat: 8g

Carbohydrates: 6g

Protein: 7g

Tender Watermelon and Radish Salad

Serving: 4

Prep Time: 15 minutes

Cook Time: 25 minutes

Ingredients:

- medium beets, peeled and cut into 1-inch chunks 1 teaspoon extra virgin olive oil 4 cups seedless watermelon, diced

- 1 tablespoon fresh thyme, chopped

- 1 lemon, juiced

- 2 cups kale, torn

- 3 cups radish, diced

- Sunflower seeds, to taste

- Pepper, to taste

How To:

1.   Pre-heat your oven to 350 degrees F.

2.   Take a small bowl and add beets, olive oil and toss well to coat the beets.

3.   Roast beets for 25 minutes until tender.

4.   Transfer to large bowl and cool them.

5.   Add watermelon, kale, radishes, thyme, lemon juice, and toss.

6.   Season sea sunflower seeds and pepper.

7.   Serve and enjoy!

Nutrition (Per Serving)

Calories: 178

Fat: 2g

Carbohydrates: 39g

Protein: 6g

Fiery Tomato Salad

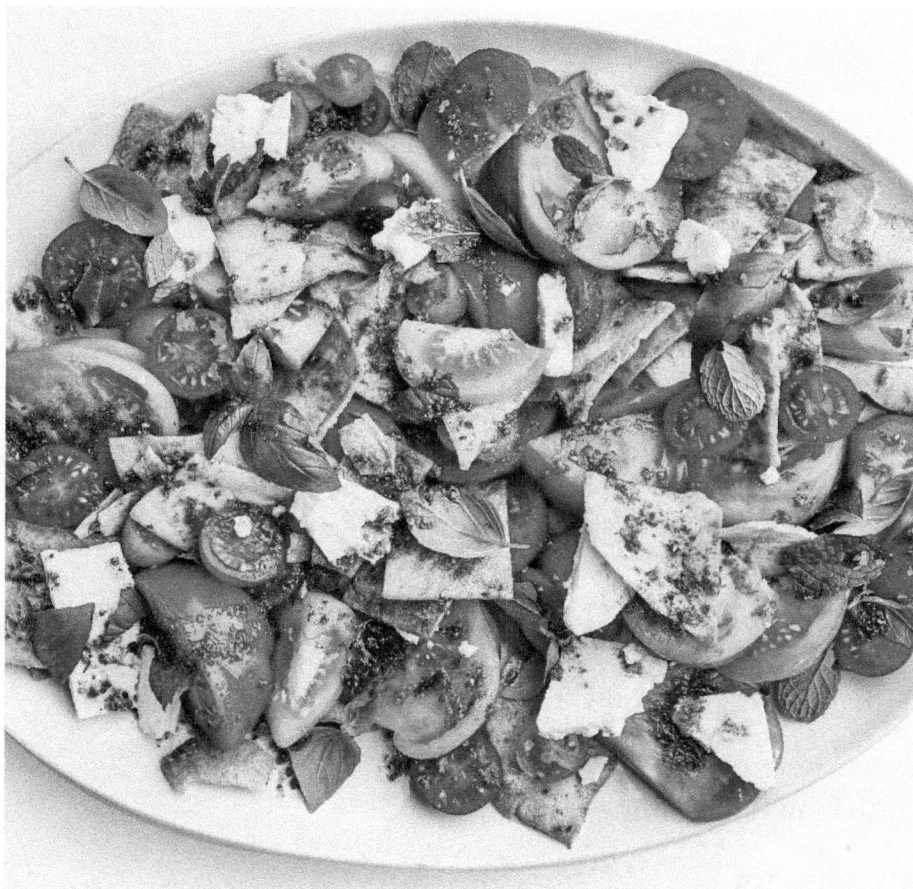

Serving: 4

Prep Time: 10 minutes

Cook Time: 25 minutes

Ingredients:

- ½ cup scallions, chopped

- 1 pound cherry tomatoes

- 3 teaspoons olive oil

- Sea sunflower seeds and freshly ground black pepper, to taste 1 tablespoon red wine vinegar

How To:

1.   Season tomatoes with spices and oil.

2.   Heat your oven to 450 degrees F.
3.   Take a baking sheet and spread the tomatoes.
4.   Bake for 15 minutes.
5.   Stir and turn the tomatoes.
6.   Then, bake again for 10 minutes.
7.   Take a bowl and mix the roasted tomatoes with all the remaining ingredients.
8.   Serve and enjoy!

Nutrition (Per Serving)

Calories: 115

Fat: 10.4g

Carbohydrates: 5.4g

Protein: 12g

Healthy Cauliflower Salad

Serving: 4

Prep Time: 10 minutes

Cook Time: nil

Ingredients:

- 1 head cauliflower, broken into florets

- 1 small onion, chopped

- 1/8 cup extra virgin olive oil

- ¼ cup apple cider vinegar

- ½ teaspoon sea salt

- ½ teaspoon black pepper

- ¼ cup dried cranberries

- ¼ cup pumpkin seeds

How To:

1. Wash the cauliflower thoroughly and break down into florets.

2. Transfer the florets to a bowl.
3. Take another bowl and whisk in oil, salt, pepper and vinegar.

4. Add pumpkin seeds, cranberries to the bowl with dressing.

5. Mix well and pour dressing over cauliflower florets.
6. Toss well.
7. Add onions and toss.
8. Chill and serve.
9. Enjoy!

Nutrition (Per Serving)

Calories: 163

Fat: 11g

Carbohydrates: 16g

Protein: 3g

Chickpea Salad

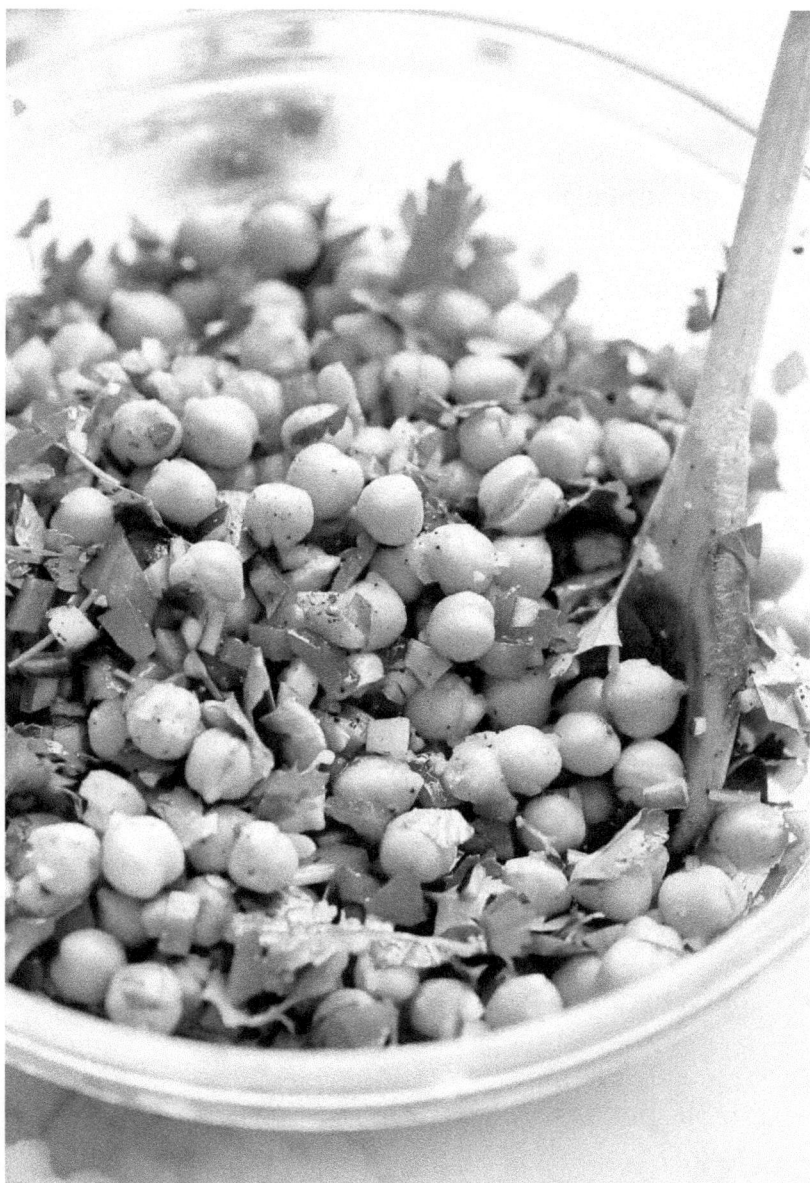

Serving: 4

Prep Time: 6 minutes

Cook Time: Nil

Ingredients:

- 1 cup canned chickpeas, drained and rinsed.

- 2 spring onions, thinly sliced.

- 1 small cucumber, diced.

- 2 green bell peppers, chopped.

- 2 tomatoes, diced.

- 2 tablespoons fresh parsley, chopped.

- 1 teaspoon capers, drained and rinsed.

- Half a lemon, juiced.

- 2 tablespoons sunflower oil.

- 1 tablespoon red wine vinegar.

- Pinch of dried oregano.

- Sunflower seeds and pepper to taste

How To:

1.   Take a medium sized bowl and add chickpeas, spring onions, cucumber, bell pepper, tomato, parsley and capers.

2.   Take another bowl and mix in the rest of the ingredients, pour mixture over chickpea salad and toss well.
3.   Coat and serve, enjoy!

Nutrition (Per Serving)

Calories: 74

Fat: 0.7g

Carbohydrates: 16g

Protein: 2g

Dashing Bok Choy Samba

Serving: 3

Prep Time: 5 minutes

Cook Time: 15 minutes

Ingredients:

- 4 bok choy, sliced

- 1 onion, sliced

- ½ cup Parmesan cheese, grated

- 4 teaspoons coconut cream

- Sunflower seeds and freshly ground black pepper, to taste

How To:

1. Mix bok choy with black pepper and sunflower seeds.

2. Take a cooking pan, heat the oil and to sauté sliced onion for 5 minutes.
3. Then add cream and seasoned bok choy.
4. Cook for 6 minutes.
5. Stir in Parmesan cheese and cover with a lid.
6. Reduce the heat to low and cook for 3 minutes.

7.   Serve warm and enjoy!

Nutrition (Per Serving)

Calories: 112

Fat: 4.9g

Carbohydrates: 1.9g

Protein: 3g

Simple Avocado Caprese Salad

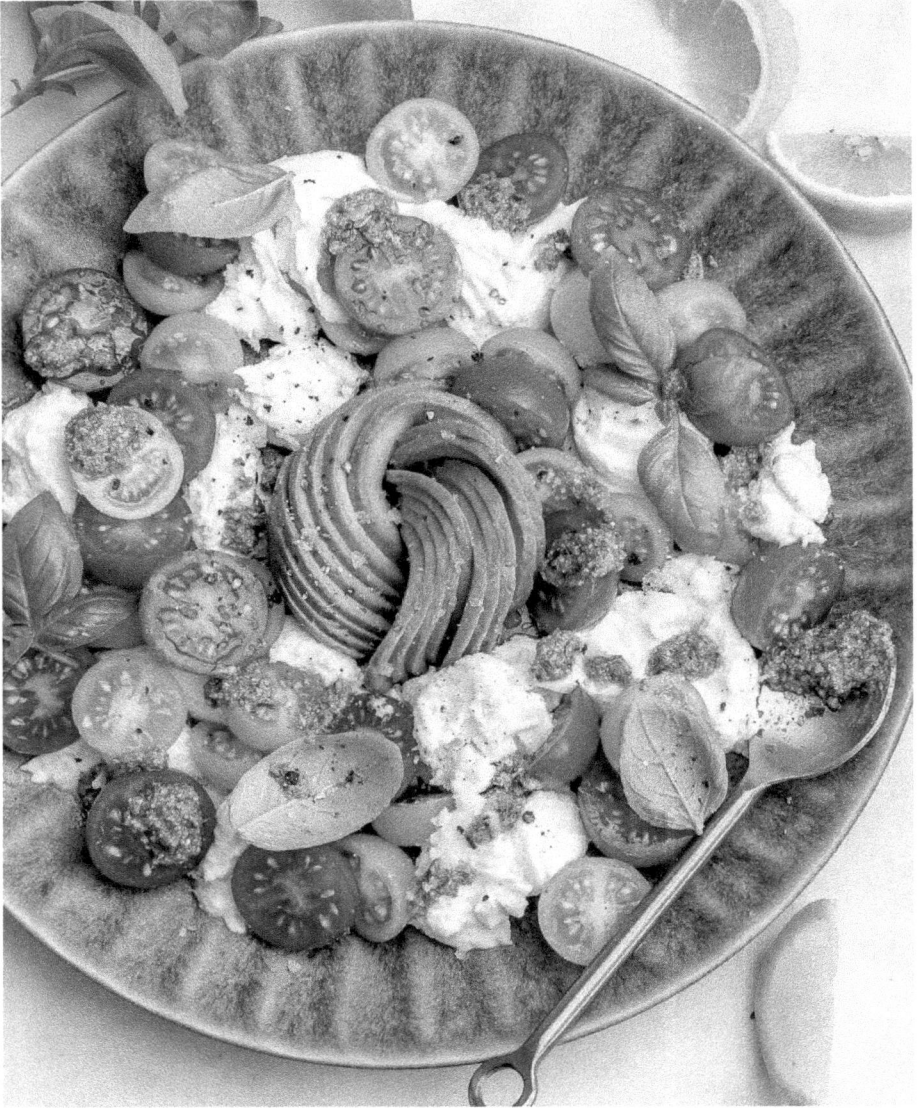

Serving: 6

Prep Time: 15 minutes

Cook Time: 29 minutes

Ingredients:

- 2 avocados, cubed

- 1 cup cherry tomatoes, halved

- 8 ounces mozzarella balls, halved

- 2 tablespoons finely chopped fresh basil

- 2 tablespoons olive oil

- 2 tablespoons balsamic vinegar

- 1 tablespoon sunflower seeds Fresh ground black pepper

How To:

1. Take a bowl and add the listed ingredients, toss them well until thoroughly mixed.

2.   Season with pepper according to your taste.

3.   Serve and enjoy!

Nutrition (Per Serving)

Calories: 358

Fat: 30g

Carbohydrates: 9g

Protein: 14g

The Rutabaga Wedge Dish

Serving: 4

Prep Time: 15 minutes

Cook Time: 45 minutes

Ingredients:

2 medium rutabagas, medium, cleaned and peeled

- 4 tablespoons almond butter

- ½ teaspoon sunflower seeds

- ½ teaspoon onion powder

- 1/8 teaspoon black pepper

- ½ cup buffalo wing sauce

- ¼ cup blue cheese dressing, low fat and low sodium 2 green onions, chopped

How To:

1.   Pre-heat your oven to 400 degrees F.

2.   Line a baking sheet with parchment paper.
3.   Wash and peel rutabagas, clean and peel them, and cut into wedge shapes.
4.   Take a skillet and place it over low heat, add almond butter and melt.
5.   Stir in onion powder, sunflower seeds, onion, black pepper.
6.   Use seasoned almond butter to coat wedges.
7.   Arrange wedges in a single layer on the baking sheet.

8.   Bake for 30 minutes.

9.   Remove and coat in buffalo sauce and return to oven.
10.   Bake for 15 minutes more.
11.   Place wedges on serving plate and trickle with blue cheese dressing.
12.   Garnish with chopped green onion and enjoy!

Nutrition (Per Serving)

Calories: 235

Fat: 15g

Carbohydrates: 10g

Protein: 2.5g

Red Coleslaw

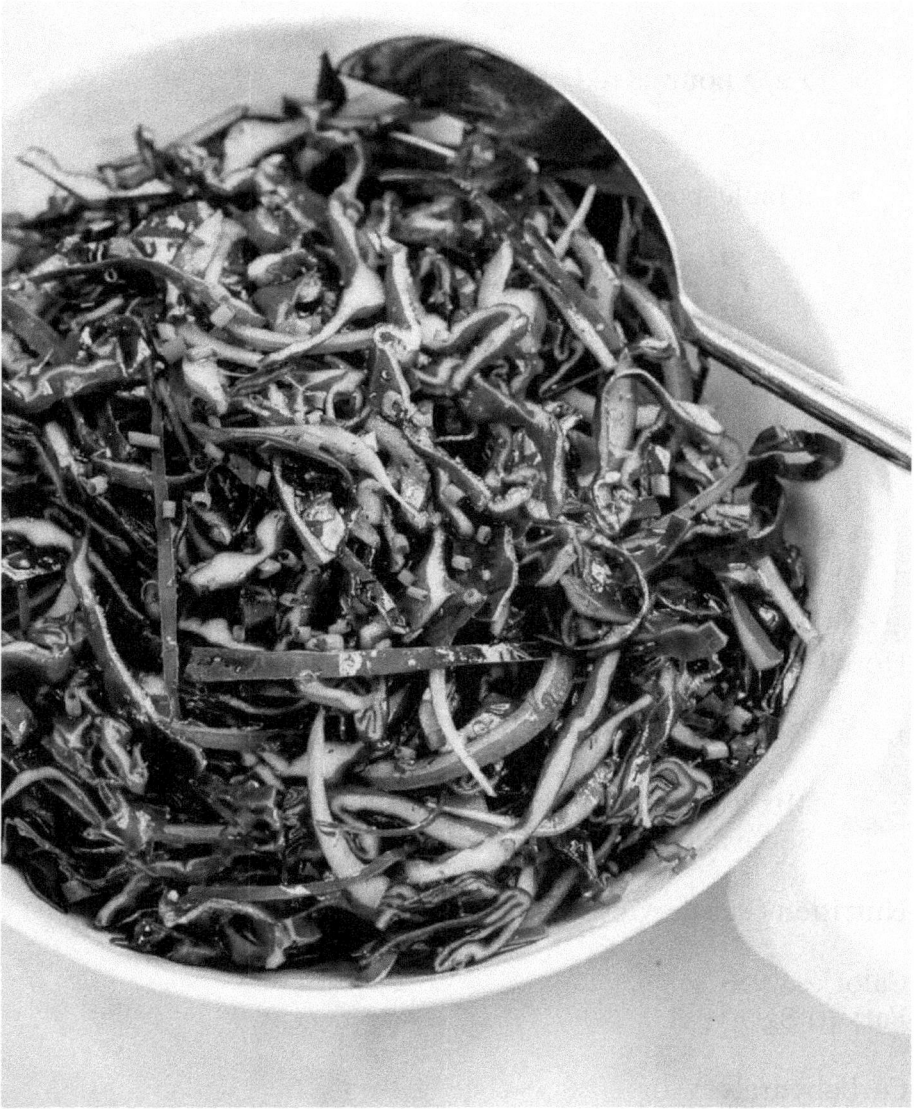

Serving: 4

Prep Time: 10 minutes

Cook Time: 0 minutes

Ingredients:

- 1 2/3 pounds red cabbage

- 2 tablespoons ground caraway seeds

- 1 tablespoon whole grain mustard

- 1 1/4 cups mayonnaise

- Sunflower seeds and black pepper

How To:

1.   Take a large bowl and all the remaining ingredients.

2.   Mix it well and let it sit for 10 minutes.
3.   Serve and enjoy!

Nutrition (Per Serving)

Calories: 406
Fat: 40.8g

Carbohydrates: 10g

Protein: 2.2g

Classic Tuna Salad

Serving: 4

Prep Time: 10 minutes

Cook Time: Nil

Ingredients:

12 ounces white tuna, in water

- ½ cup celery, diced

- 2 tablespoons fresh parsley, chopped

- 2 tablespoons low-calorie mayonnaise, low fat and low sodium

- ½ teaspoon Dijon mustard

- ½ teaspoon sunflower seeds

- ¼ teaspoon fresh ground black pepper

Direction

1.   Take a medium sized bowl and add tuna, parsley, and celery.

2. Mix well and add mayonnaise and mustard.
3. Season with pepper and sunflower seeds.
4. Stir and add olives, relish, chopped pickle, onion and mix well.

5. Serve and enjoy

Nutrition (Per Serving)

Calories: 137

Fat: 5g

Carbohydrates: 1g

Protein: 20g

Greek Salad

Serving: 4

Prep Time: 6 minutes

Cook Time: Nil

Ingredients:

- 2 cucumbers, diced

- 2 tomatoes, sliced

- 1 green lettuce, cut into thin strips

- 2 red bell peppers, cut

- ½ cup black olives pitted

- 3 ½ ounces feta cheese, cut

- 1 red onion, sliced

- 2 tablespoons olive oil

- 2 tablespoons lemon juice

- Sunflower seeds and pepper to taste

Direction

1.　　Dice cucumbers and slice up the tomatoes.

2.　　Tear the lettuce and cut it into thin strips.
3.　　De-seed and cut the peppers into strips.
4.　　Take a salad bowl and mix in all the listed vegetables, add olives and feta cheese (cut into cubes).
5.　　Take a small cup and mix in olive oil and lemon juice, season with sunflower seeds and pepper.
6.　　Pour mixture into the salad and toss well, enjoy!

Nutrition (Per Serving)

Calories: 132

Fat: 4g

Carbohydrates: 3g

Protein: 5g

Fancy Greek Orzo Salad

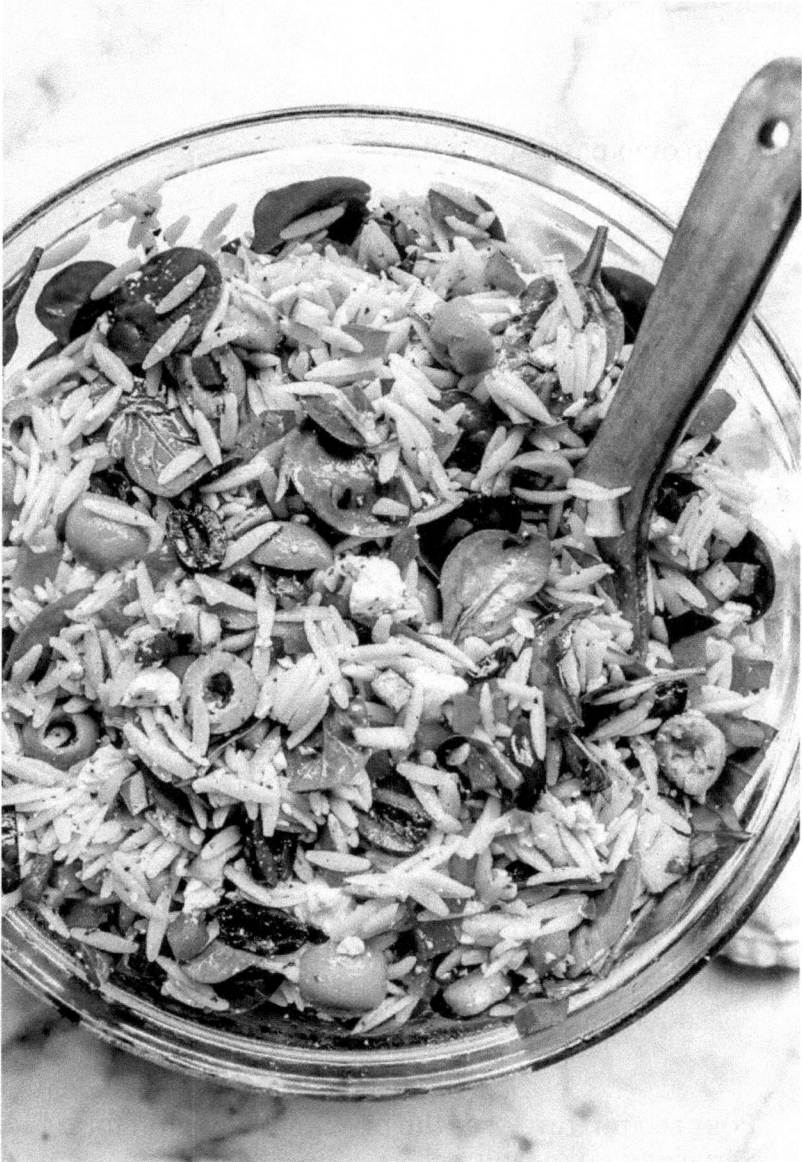

Serving: 4

Prep Time: 5 minutes and 24 hours chill time

Cook Time: 10 minutes

Ingredients:

- 1 cup orzo pasta, uncooked

- ½ cup fresh parsley, minced

- 6 teaspoons olive oil

- 1 onion, chopped

- 1 ½ teaspoons oregano

How To:

1.   Cook the orzo and drain them.

2.   Add to a serving dish.
3.   Add 2 teaspoons of oil.
4.   Take another dish and add parsley, onion, remaining oil and oregano.
5.   Season with sunflower seeds, pepper according to your taste.

6.   Pour the mixture over the orzo and let it chill for 24 hours.
7.   Serve and enjoy at lunch!

Nutrition (Per Serving)

Calories: 399

Fat: 12g

Carbohydrates: 55g

Protein:16g

Homely Tuscan Tuna Salad

Serving: 4

Prep Time: 5-10 minutes

Cook Time: Nil

Ingredients:

- 15 ounces small white beans

- 6 ounces drained chunks of light tuna

- cherry tomatoes, quartered

- 4 scallions, trimmed and sliced

- 2 tablespoons lemon juice

How To:

Add all of the listed ingredients to a bowl and gently stir.

Season with sunflower seeds and pepper accordingly, enjoy!

Nutrition (Per Serving)

Calories: 322

Fat: 8g

Carbohydrates: 32g

Protein:30g

Asparagus Loaded Lobster Salad

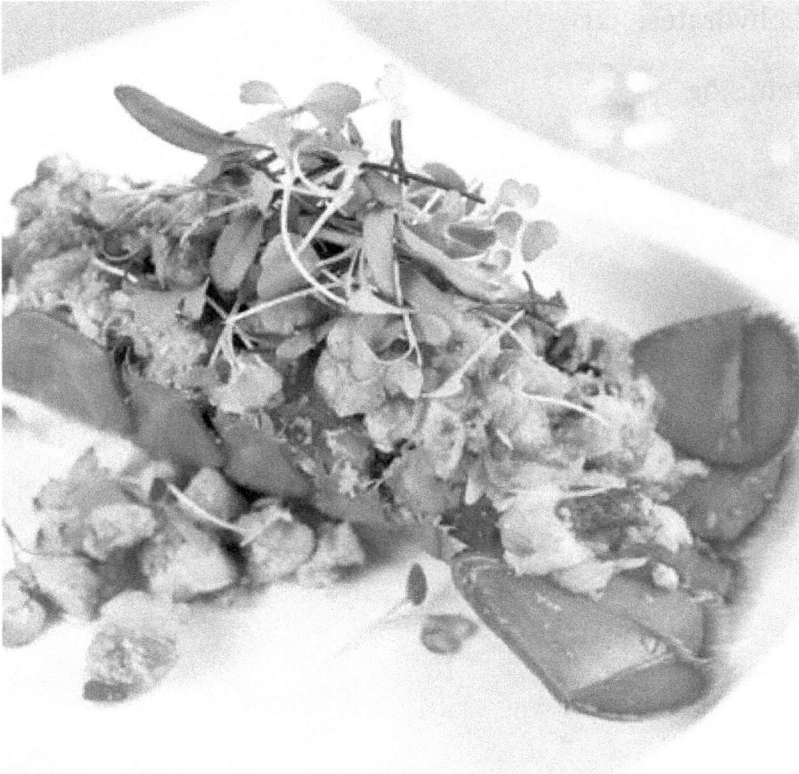

Serving: 4

Prep Time: 10 minutes

Cook Time: Nil

Ingredients:

- 8 ounces lobster, cooked and chopped

- 3 ½ cups asparagus, chopped and steamed

- 2 tablespoons lemon juice

- 4 teaspoons extra virgin olive oil

- ¼ teaspoon kosher sunflower seeds

- Pepper

- ½ cup cherry tomatoes halved

- 1 basil leaf, chopped

- 2 tablespoons red onion, diced

How To:

1.   Whisk in lemon juice, sunflower seeds, pepper in a bowl and mix with oil.

2.   Take a bowl and add the rest of the ingredients.
3.   Toss well and pour dressing on top.

Serve and enjoy!

Nutrition (Per Serving)

Calories: 247

Fat: 10g

Carbohydrates: 14g

Protein: 27g

Tasty Yogurt and Cucumber Salad

Serving: 4

Prep Time: 10 minutes

Cook Time: Nil

Ingredients:

- 5-6 small cucumbers, peeled and diced

- 1 (8 ounces) container plain Greek yogurt

- 2 garlic cloves, minced

- 1 tablespoon fresh mint, minced

- Sea sunflower seeds and fresh black pepper

How To:

Take a large bowl and add cucumbers, garlic, yogurt, mint.

Season with sunflower seeds and pepper.

Refrigerate the salad for 1 hour and serve.

Enjoy!

Nutrition (Per Serving)

Calories: 74

Fat: 0.7g

Carbohydrates: 16g

Protein: 2g

Unique Eggplant Salad

Serving: 3

Prep Time: 10 minutes

Cook Time: 30 minutes

Ingredients:

2 eggplants, peeled and sliced

- 2 garlic cloves

- 2 green bell pepper, sliced, seeds removed ½ cup fresh parsley

- ½ cup mayonnaise, low fat, low sodium Sunflower seeds and black pepper

How To:

1.   Preheat your oven to 480 degrees F.

2.   Take a baking pan and add eggplant, bell peppers and season with black [MOU15][F16]pepper to it.
3.   Bake for about 30 minutes.
4.   Flip the vegetables after 20 minutes.
5.   Then, take a bowl, add baked vegetables and all the remaining ingredients.
6.   Mix well.
7.   Serve and enjoy!

Nutrition (Per Serving)

Calories: 196

Fat: 108.g

Carbohydrates: 13.4g

Protein: 14.6g

Zucchini Pesto Salad

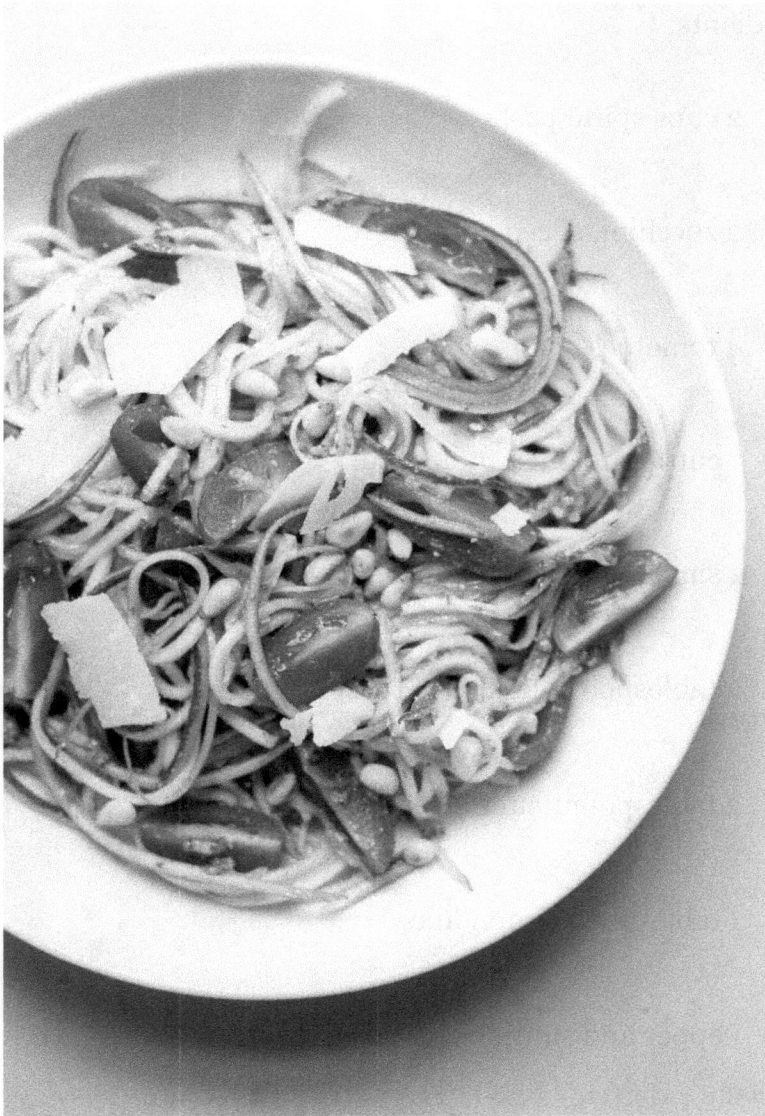

Serving: 4

Prep Time: 10 minutes

Cook Time: 10 minutes

Ingredients:

- 2 cups spiral pasta

- 2 zucchini, sliced and halved

- 4 tomatoes, cut

- 1 cup white mushrooms, cut

- 1 small red onion, chopped

- 2 tablespoons fresh basil leaves, chopped

- 2 tablespoons sunflower oil

- 1 tablespoon lemon juice

- Pepper and sunflower seeds to taste

How To:

1.   Cook the pasta according to the package instructions, drain and rinse under cold water.

2.	Take a large bowl and add zucchini, tomatoes, mushrooms, onion, and pasta.
3.	Mix well,
4.	In a food processor, add oil, lemon juice, basil, blue cheese, black, and process well.
5.	Pour the mixture over the salad and toss well.
6.	Serve and enjoy!

Nutrition (Per Serving)

Calories: 301

Fat: 25g

Net Carbohydrates: 7g

Protein: 10g

Wholesome Potato and Tuna Salad

Serving: 4

Prep Time: 10 minutes

Cook Time: nil

Ingredients:

- 1 pound baby potatoes, scrubbed, boiled

- 1 cup tuna chunks, drained

- 1 cup cherry tomatoes, halved

- 1 cup medium onion, thinly sliced

- 8 pitted black olives

- 2 medium hard-boiled eggs, sliced

- 1 head Romaine lettuce

- ¼ cup olive oil

- 2 tablespoons lemon juice

- 1 tablespoon Dijon mustard

- 1 teaspoon dill weed, chopped Pepper as needed

How To:

1.   Take a small glass bowl and mix in your olive oil, lemon juice, Dijon mustard and dill.

2.   Season the mix with pepper and salt.
3.   Add in the tuna, baby potatoes, cherry tomatoes, red onion, green beans, black olives and toss everything nicely.
4.   Arrange your lettuce leaves on a beautiful serving dish to make the base of your salad.
5.   Top them with your salad mixture and place the egg slices.
6.   Drizzle with the previously prepared Salad Dressing.
7.   Serve hot

Nutrition (Per Serving)

Calories: 406

Fat: 22g

Carbohydrates: 28g

Protein: 26g

Baby Spinach Salad

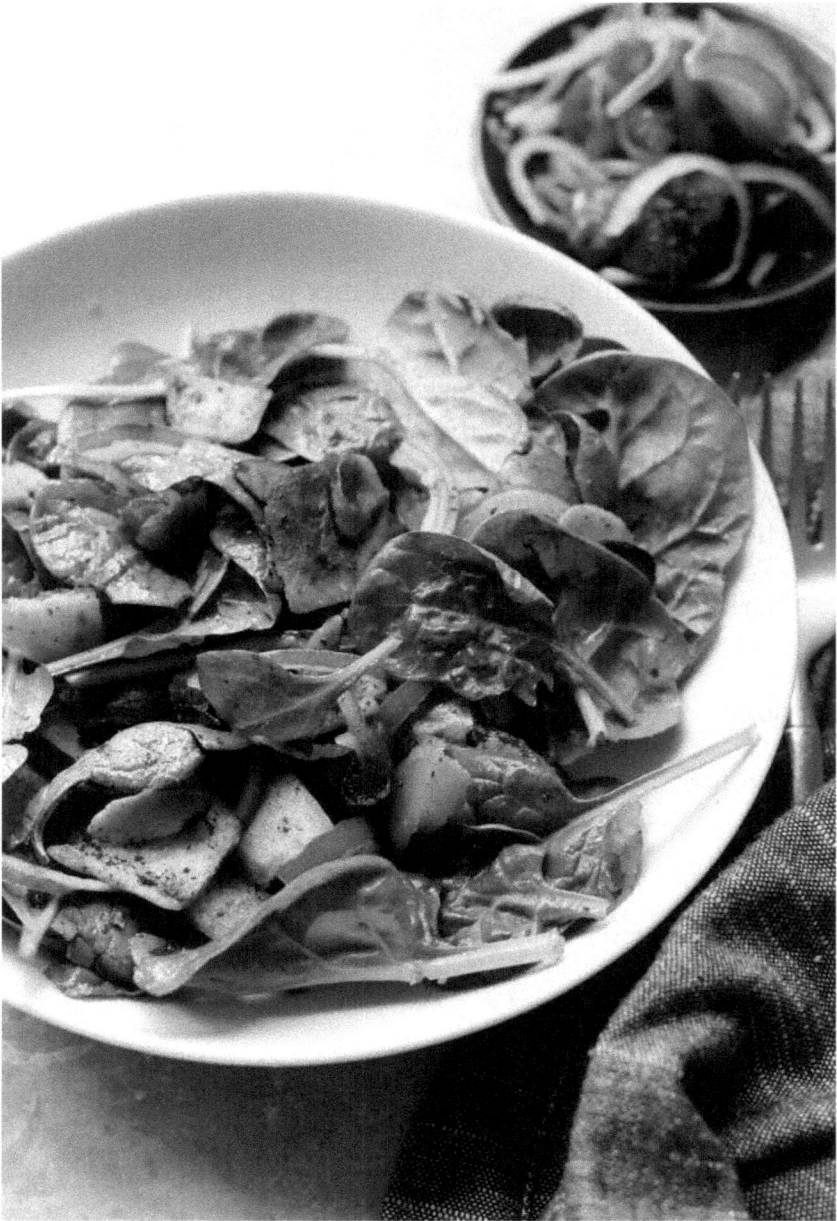

Serving: 2

Prep Time: 10 minutes

Cook Time: nil

Ingredients:

- 1 bag baby spinach, washed and dried

- 1 red bell pepper, cut in slices

- 1 cup cherry tomatoes, cut in halves

- 1 small red onion, finely chopped

- 1 cup black olives, pitted

For dressing:

- 1 teaspoon dried oregano

- 1 large garlic clove

- 3 tablespoons red wine vinegar

- 4 tablespoons olive oil

- Sunflower seeds and pepper to taste

How To:

1.   Prepare the dressing by blending in garlic, olive oil, vinegar in a food processor.

2.   Take a large salad bowl and add spinach leaves, toss well with the dressing.
3.   Add remaining ingredients and toss again, season with sunflower seeds and pepper and enjoy!

Nutrition (Per Serving)

Calories: 126

Fat: 10g

Carbohydrates: 10g

Protein: 2g

Elegant Corn Salad

Serving: 6

Prep Time: 10 minutes

Cooking Time: 2 hours

Ingredients:

- 2 ounces prosciutto, cut into strips

- 1 teaspoon olive oil

- 2 cups corn

- 1/2 cup salt-free tomato sauce

- 1 teaspoon garlic, minced

- 1 green bell pepper, chopped

How To:

1. Grease your Slow Cooker with oil.

2.   Add corn, prosciutto, garlic, tomato sauce, bell pepper to your Slow Cooker.

3.   Stir and place lid.
4.   Cook on HIGH for 2 hours.
5.   Divide between serving platters and enjoy!

Nutrition (Per Serving)

Calories: 109

Fat: 2g

Carbohydrates: 10g

Protein: 5g

Arabic Fattoush Salad

Serving: 4

Prep Time: 15 minutes

Cook Time: 2-3 minutes

Ingredients:

- 1 whole wheat pita bread

- 1 large English cucumber, diced

- 2 cup grape tomatoes, halved

- ½ medium red onion, finely diced

- ¾ cup fresh parsley, chopped

- ¾ cup mint leaves, chopped

- 1 clove garlic, minced

- ¼ cup fat free feta cheese, crumbled

- 1 tablespoon olive oil

- 1 teaspoon ground sumac

- Juice from ½ a lemon

- Salt and pepper as needed

How To:

1. Mist pita bread with cooking spray.
2. Season with salt.
3. Toast until the breads are crispy.

4. Take a large bowl and add the remaining ingredients and mix (except feta).

5. Top the mix with diced toasted pita and feta.
6. Serve and enjoy!

Nutrition (Per Serving)

Calories: 86

Fat: 3g

Carbohydrates: 9g

Protein: 9g

Heart Warming Cauliflower Salad

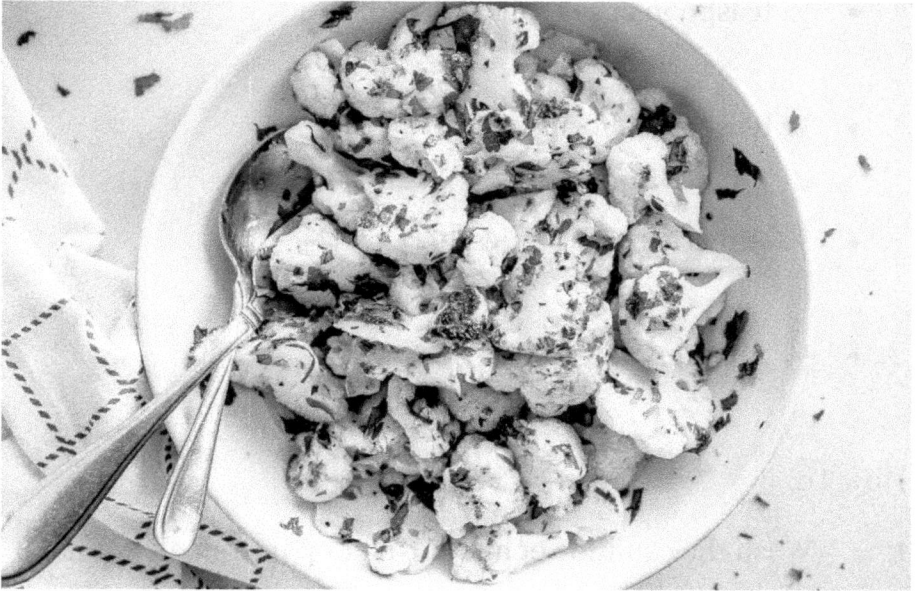

Serving: 3

Prep Time: 8 minutes

Cook Time: nil

Ingredients:

- 1 head cauliflower, broken into florets

- 1 small onion, chopped

- 1/8 cup extra virgin olive oil

- ¼ cup apple cider vinegar

- ½ teaspoon of sea salt

- ½ teaspoon of black pepper

- ¼ cup dried cranberries

- ¼ cup pumpkin seeds

How To:

1. Wash the cauliflower and break it up into small florets.

2. Transfer to a bowl.
3. Whisk oil, vinegar, salt and pepper in another bowl.
4. Add pumpkin seeds, cranberries to the bowl with dressing.
5. Mix well and pour the dressing over the cauliflower.
6. Add onions and toss.
7. Chill and serve.
8. Enjoy!

Nutrition (Per Serving)

Calories: 163

Fat: 11g

Carbohydrates: 16g

Protein: 3g

Great Greek Sardine Salad

Serving: 2

Prep Time: 10 minutes

Cook Time: 10 minutes

Ingredients:

- 2 tablespoons extra virgin olive oil

- 1 garlic clove, minced

- 2 teaspoons dried oregano

- ½ teaspoon freshly ground pepper

- 3 medium tomatoes, cut into large sized chunks

- 1 can (15 ounces) rinsed chickpeas

- 1/3 cup feta cheese, crumbled

- ¼ cup red onion, sliced

- 2 tablespoons Kalamata olives, sliced

- 2 cans 4-ounce drained sardines, with bones and packed in either oil or water

How To:

1.   Take a large bowl and whisk in lemon juice, oregano, garlic, oil, pepper and mix well.

2.   Add tomatoes, chickpeas, cucumber, olives, feta and mix.
3.   Divide the salad amongst serving platter and top with sardines.

4.   Enjoy!

Nutrition (Per Serving)

Calories: 347

Fat: 18g

Carbohydrates: 29g

Protein: 17g

Shrimp and Egg Medley

Serving: 4

Prep Time: 15 minutes

Cook Time: nil

Ingredients:

- 4 hard boiled eggs, peeled and chopped

- 1 pound cooked shrimp, peeled and deveined, chopped

- 1 sprig fresh dill, chopped

- ¼ cup mayonnaise

- 1 teaspoon Dijon mustard

- 4 fresh lettuce leaves

How To:

1.   Take a large serving bowl and add the listed ingredients (except lettuce).

2.   Stir well.
3.   Serve over bed of lettuce leaves.

4.   Enjoy!

Nutrition (Per Serving)

Calories: 292

Fat: 17g

Carbohydrates: 1.6g

Protein: 30g

Creamy Shrimp Salad

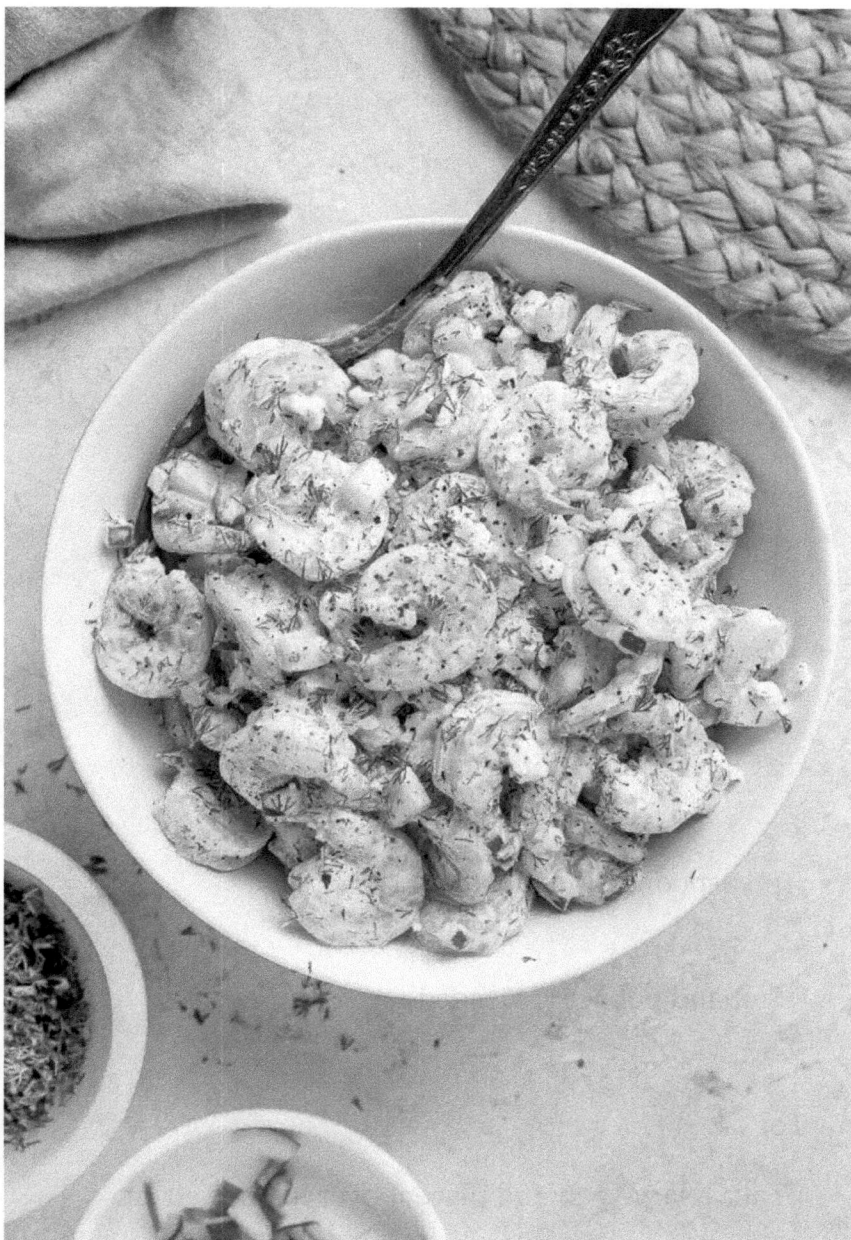

Serving: 4

Prep Time: 20 minutes

Cook Time: 5 minutes

Ingredients:

- 4 pounds large shrimp

- 1 lemon, quartered

- 3 cups celery stalks, chopped

- 1 red onion, chopped

- 2 cups mayonnaise

- 2 tablespoons white wine vinegar

- 1 teaspoon Dijon mustard

- Salt and pepper as needed

How To:

1.   Take a large pan and place it over medium heat.

2.   Add water (salted) and bring water to boil.
3.   Add shrimp and lemon, cook for 3 minutes.

4.   Let them cool.
5.   Peel and de-vein the shrimps.
6.   Take a large bowl and add cooked shrimp alongside remaining ingredients.
7.   Stir well.
8.   Serve immediately or chilled!

Nutrition (Per Serving)

Calories: 153

Fat: 5g

Carbohydrates: 8g

Protein: 19g

Passionate Quinoa and Black Bean Salad

Serving: 6

Prep Time: 5 minutes

Cook Time: 15 minutes

Ingredients:

- 1 cup uncooked quinoa

- 1 can 15 ounce black beans, drained and rinsed 1/3 cup cilantro, chopped

- 1 tablespoon olive oil

- 1 clove garlic, minced

- Juice from 1 lime

- Salt and pepper as needed

How To:

1.   Cook quinoa according to the package instructions.

2.   Transfer quinoa to a medium bowl and let it cool for 10 minutes.

3.   Add remaining ingredients and toss well.
4.   Serve and enjoy!

Nutrition (Per Serving)

Calories: 188

Fat: 4g

Carbohydrates: 29g

Protein: 8g

Zucchini Noodle Salad

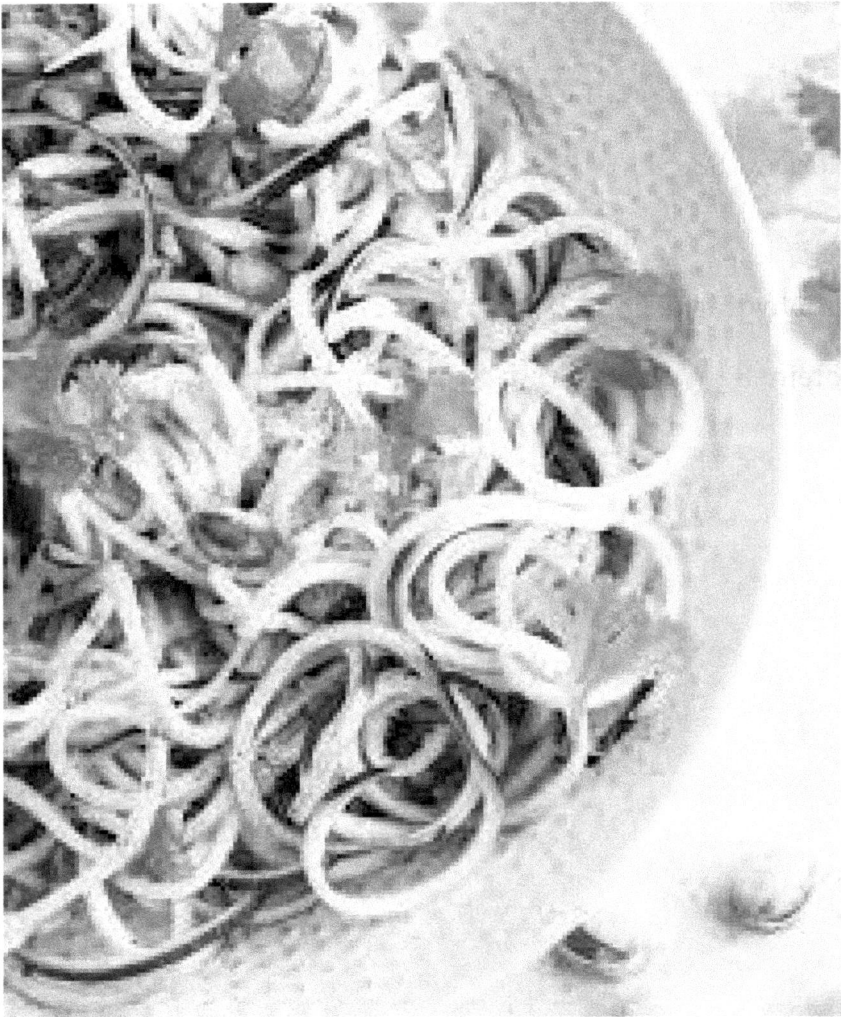

Serving: 3

Prep Time: 15 minutes

Cook Time: nil

Ingredients:

- 2 large zucchini, spiralized/peeled into thin strips

- 1 small tomato, diced

- ¼ red onion, sliced thinly

- 1 large avocado, diced

- ½ cup olive oil
- ¼ cup balsamic vinegar

- 1 garlic clove, minced

- 2 teaspoons Dijon mustard

- Salt and pepper to taste

- ¼ cup blue cheese, crumbles

How To:

1.	Take a large bowl and add zucchini noodles, onion, tomato, avocado.

2.	Take a small bowl and whisk in olive oil, vinegar, mustard, garlic, salt and pepper.
3.	Drizzle over salad and toss.

4.   Divide into serving bowls and top with blue cheese crumbles.

5.   Enjoy!

Nutrition (Per Serving)

Calories: 770

Fat: 74g

Carbohydrates: 12g

Protein: 8g

www.ingramcontent.com/pod-product-compliance
Lightning Source LLC
Chambersburg PA
CBHW070722030426

42336CB00013B/1888